CLINICIAN'S GUIDE

The Dentist's Role in the Management of the Cancer Patient

Editors	Contents	Pg

Wendy S. Hupp, D.M.D.
Assistant Professor of Oral Medicine
Department of General Dentistry and Oral Medicine
University of Louisville School of Dentistry
Louisville, Kentucky

Cesar Augusto Migliorati D.D.S., M.S., Ph.D.
Professor and Director- Oral Medicine
Department of Biologic & Diagnostic Sciences
University of Tennessee Health Science Center
College of Dentistry
Memphis, Tennessee

Mike Brennan D.D.S., M.H.S.
Associate Chairman & Director, Sjögren's Syndrome and Salivary Disorders Center
Department of Oral Medicine
Carolinas Medical Center
Charlotte, North Carolina

Contributing Authors

Norbert J. Burzynski, Sr., D.D.S., M.S.

F. John Firriolo, D.D.S., Ph.D.

Craig Hatch, D.M.D.

Michaell A. Huber, D.D.S.

Barbara A. Murphy, M.D.

Contributing authors are members of the American Academy of Oral Medicine. This monograph represents a consensus of the contributing authors and not necessarily the private views of any of the individuals

Contents Pg

American Academy of Oral Medicine
23607 Hwy 99, Suite 2C
Edmonds, WA 98026-9272
Tel: (425) 778-6162
Fax: (425) 771-9588
Email: info@aaom.com
www.aaom.com

ISBN [print]: 978-1-936-176-12-0
Printed in the United States

Notice: The authors and publisher have made every effort to ensure that the patient care recommended herein, including choice of drugs and drug dosages, is in accord with the accepted standard and practice at the time of publication. However, since research and regulation constantly change clinical standards, the reader is urged to check the product information sheet included in the package of each drug, which includes recommended doses, warnings, and contraindications. This is particularly important with new or infrequently used drugs. Any treatment regimen, particularly one involving medication, involves inherent risk that must be weighed on a case-by-case basis against the benefits anticipated. The reader is cautioned that the purpose of this book is to inform and enlighten; the information contained herein is not intended as, and should not be employed as, a substitute for individual diagnosis and treatment.

The first edition of this Guide is dedicated to the memory of Jonathan A. Ship, DMD. Dr. Ship was an inspiration to a generation of students, oral medicine residents and colleagues and a revered member of the American Academy of Oral Medicine. His research contributions in geriatric dentistry, xerostomia, Sjögren's syndrome and oral, head and neck cancer will serve the professional community and society for generations. His friendship, guidance, professionalism and laughter are sorely missed by everyone who knew and loved him. Dr. Ship has contributed extensively to this Guide.

ABOUT THE AMERICAN ACADEMY OF ORAL MEDICINE (AAOM) - The AAOM is a 501c6, nonprofit organization founded in 1945 as the American Academy of Dental Medicine and took its current name in 1966. The members of the American Academy of Oral Medicine include an internationally recognized group of health care professionals and experts concerned with the oral health care of patients who have complex medical conditions, oral mucosal disorders, and / or chronic orofacial pain. Oral Medicine is the field of dentistry concerned with the oral health care of medically complex patients and with the diagnosis and non-surgical management of medically-related disorders or conditions affecting the oral and maxillofacial region.

The American Academy of Oral Medicine • *(425) 778-6162* • *www.aaom.com* • *23607 Hwy 99, Suite 2C* • *Edmonds, WA• 98026-9272*

AMERICAN ACADEMY OF ORAL MEDICINE

Mission:

1. To promote the study and dissemination of knowledge of the medical aspects of dentistry while serving the best interests of the public.
2. To promote the highest standards of care in the diagnosis and treatment of oral conditions that are not responsive to conventional dental or oral maxillofacial surgical procedures.
3. To provide an avenue of referral for dental practitioners who have patients with severe, life-threatening medical disorders or complex diagnostic problems involving the oral and maxillofacial region that require ongoing nonsurgical management.
4. To improve the quality of life of patients with medically related oral disease.
5. To foster increased understanding and cooperation between medical and dental professions.
6. To obtain American Dental Association recognition of oral medicine as a specialty.

The Academy achieves these goals by holding national meetings annually; by presenting lectures, workshops, and seminars; by sponsorship of the American Board of Oral Medicine; by the editorship of the Oral Medicine Section of *Oral Surgery, Oral Medicine, Oral Pathology, Oral Radiology and Endodontics*; and by publishing monographs and position papers on timely subjects relating to oral medicine.

The presented information is based on current knowledge and accepted standards of practice. Following the guidelines set forth in this monograph may not ensure successful management of every patient. This monograph represents a consensus of the editors and authors and not necessarily the private views of any individual.

All brand name medications may have patents, service marks, trademarks, or registered trademarks and are the property of their respective companies.

This *Clinician's Guide* is another AAOM educational service. Other Clinician's Guides available from the Academy include:

Treatment of Common Oral Conditions, 7/e
Tobacco Cessation, 2/e
Oral Health in Geriatric Patients, 3/e
Pharmacology, 2/e
Diagnosis and Treatment of Chronic Orofacial Pain, 3/e
Medically Complex Dental Patients, 4/e
Salivary Gland & Chemosensory Disorders
Diagnosis of Oral Cancer and Potentially Malignant Lesions

INTRODUCTION

Cancer is one of the leading causes of death within the United States (see below). Dentist within the United States will, as a routine part of practice, see patients who have cancer and are under the care of the oncologist, or who survived cancer. The aggressive use of combined modality treatment approaches, novel drug therapies and the use of high dose therapy with stem cell transplantation have led to an increased number of cancer survivors. Although novel and aggressive therapies have successfully improved survival, they have done so at the expense of increased rates of both acute and late toxicities. Oral health complications of treatment are common but understudied and under appreciate treatment effects that can lead to substantial morbidity, and in severe cases, can limit cancer therapy and affect prognosis. It is therefore critical for Dentist and other health professionals to become an active and integral member of the Oncology treatment team. In order to do so, it is imperative that all Oral Health Care providers familiarize themselves with general principles of cancer, cancer therapy and the adverse oral health outcomes that need to be addressed. Although most dentists are comfortable with the diagnosis and management of patients with oral cancers, they may feel uncomfortable treating patients with other malignancies.

Cancer Facts:

- 1 in 2 males will develop cancer of some type in their lifetime. 1 in 4 will die.
- 1 in 3 females will develop cancer of some type in their lifetimes. 1 in 5 will die.
- 11 million Americans with a history of cancer were alive in January 2006.
- About 1,473,350 new cancer cases were expected to be diagnosed in 2009.
- 1 in 209 people in the U.S. will develop cancer this year.
- 5 year survival rate for all cancers diagnosed between 1999 and 2005 is 69% (up from 55% for 1975-1977).
- 562,340 patients were expected to die of cancer in 2009.
- Cancer accounts for 1 in 4 deaths in the U.S.

This monograph was written with the goal of familiarizing Dentists with current cancer therapies and how they impact oral health. It will also discuss the medical and dental management with a focus on the care of cancer patients who need oral/dental care for stabilization of oral health prior, during cancer therapy that might adversely affect the oral mucosa, teeth and periodontium, and after therapy when management of chronic adverse effects is of critical importance. The management principles are similar to those discussed previously in the *AAOM Clinicians Guide to Diagnosis of Oral Cancer and Potentially Malignant Oral Lesions*. Since the topic "oral cancer care" was recently reviewed, it will be omitted from this monograph.

How does this relate to a typical practice?

Practitioners frequently ask if oral care for cancer patients is a sufficiently common clinical scenario to merit ongoing education or special attention. The answer is clearly ***yes***. For sake of discussion, assume that a practice has 1,000 patients. In a given year, you would expect to see 5 patients with newly diagnosed cancer and 37 cancer survivors. The number of survivors is likely to increase as cancer therapy increases the rate of cure and the length of survival.

- 5 new cancer cases per year
- 37 patients with a history of cancer
- 8 patients with a history of breast cancer
- 7 patients with a history of prostate cancer.
- 1 patient with a history of lung cancer
- 4 patients with a history of genital system cancer
- 3 patients with a history of leukemia, lymphoma and multiple myeloma
- 4 patients with history of colon and rectal cancer

Dentists are part of the cancer management team.

The management of a patient with cancer requires a team approach. In general, the treatment plan for cancer patients is discussed at hospital based *tumor boards*. A tumor board is composed of professionals with expertise in oncologic surgery, chemotherapy, radiation therapy, dentistry and maxillofacial prosthodontics, radiology, pathology, nutritionists, social workers, and counselors. In the ideal case:

- All members of the team meet to discuss the best management of the patient with cancer
- All members of the team have equal access to all the diagnostic information, staging, and psychological evaluation
- The treatment options and prognosis of each are openly discussed and agreed upon
- All members of the team have input to the best treatment course for each particular patient
- This recommended best treatment course is presented to the patient for their approval

Therefore, in order to provide the most appropriate oral care for cancer patients, the dentist should be an integral member of this cancer management team. In most instances, however, dentists are not working in hospitals or cancer centers. Patients are referred to their family dentist for a pre cancer treatment evaluation. Often dentists who are not working in close collaboration with the cancer treatment center will find it difficult to access all the diagnostic information on the patient, to understand the expected oral toxicities from each modality of treatment, and to understand the physician's patient assessment.

It therefore becomes the responsibility of the Dentist to communicate with the other members of the Oncology Team. More often than not, Oral Health Professionals need to educate the other members of the Oncology Team about the role of dental professions in the care of cancer patients. Listed below is a list of objectives for Oral Health Providers to use when treating cancer patients.

- Diagnose and treat oral disease prior to the starting of cancer therapy whenever possible
- Establish a proper oral hygiene protocol that will help the patient to maintain oral health before, during and after cancer therapy
- Establish a baseline for comparison and monitoring sequelae of radiation and chemotherapy damage
- Diagnose and manage oral complications of cancer therapy
- Detect metastatic or recurrent lesions
- Minimize oral discomfort and maintain function of the oral cavity for proper nutrition during and after cancer treatment
- Communicate with the Oncology Team when referrals to other specialists is indicated: for example – nutrition consultation for weight loss due to dental issues, physical therapy for trismus, speech and swallowing therapists for patients with dysphagia

Defining the Scope of the Problem.

In order to effectively diagnose, prevent and treat oral complications of cancer therapy, the Oral Health Professional must have a working knowledge of the potential impact of cancer and cancer therapy on oral health. Oral complications related to cancer treatment are common (see Table 1). By anticipating these problems and educating the patient and the family members on what to expect, the cancer treatment may be more easily tolerated, leading to improved outcomes of therapy and the quality of life of the patient.

Table 1 Oral Complications of Cancer Treatment	
Cancer Treatment Regimen	**% of patients with oral complications**
Head and neck radiation therapy that includes the salivary glands	**100**
Hematopoietic stem cell transplant	**80**
Chemotherapy (primary)	**40**
Adjuvant chemotherapy or immunotherapy	**10**

How to use this monograph:

This monograph is organized into five sections. The first section reviews general principles of cancer therapy. The next three sections discuss how the dentist should evaluate and treat cancer patients at differing stages in the trajectory of their disease. Finally, the fifth section will review the complications of cancer therapy and describe treatment for these complications.

Section 1 - Basics of Cancer Therapy

Section 2 - Dental Considerations Prior to Cancer Treatment

Section 3 - Dental Considerations During Cancer Treatment

Section 4 - Dental Considerations Post Cancer Treatment

Section 5 - Oral complications and Treatment

Unfortunately, most patients are not referred for dental evaluation prior to initiating cancer therapy. Furthermore, continuity of dental care is frequently lacking. It is therefore likely that Oral Health Professionals will do an initial assessment of patients who are either in active treatment or have completed cancer therapy. In each case, understanding the implications of response to cancer therapy, risk of tumor recurrence, and expected patient survival are important when designing a treatment plan. Review the section on the patient's current disease stage to find related information.

Wendy S. Hupp, Cesar Augusto Migliorati, and Mike Brennan, Editors.

1 – Basics of Cancer Therapy

History

Medical and Dental History

All patients with cancer who are planned for therapeutic interventions that include chemotherapy or radiation therapy to the head and neck should undergo a thorough medical and dental history. At the time of diagnosis, patients are often overwhelmed. Dental assessment and care may seem a trivial issue at this stressful point in the patient's life. It is important for the oral health care team to work with the patient in order to obtain information needed to guide treatment recommendations. In addition, cancer patients often have significant comorbidities which may seem minor to them at the time. Patients must be carefully queried about chronic diseases that may further impact on treatment recommendations.

In addition to medical issues, it is important to assess social and financial barriers to oral health care. Patients are often concerned about transportation, scheduling multiple appointments in a short time frame, and burden on family and friends. These concerns may sway them to forgo needed oral care. Helping patients to understand the importance of oral care in the near and long term is a critical role for oral health providers. In addition, working with patients to ensure timely appointments that fit into their overall treatment schedule can be helpful and reassuring. Finally, patients are often concerned about the cost of care. This is particularly problematic for the patient who is the "bread winner" for the family and is facing temporary or permanent loss of income. In developing a dental treatment plan, the Oral Health Professional must thoroughly assess the patient's medical and dental history.

- Medical History
  - All diseases and conditions under medical care, including the cancer. It is important to know the type of cancer, the staging, the planned cancer therapy and expected oral toxicities
  - List of medications, dosage and duration of therapy
  - A list of allergies and adverse reactions to medications
  - When the cancer treatment is scheduled to start
  - Planned course of cancer treatment
  - Name and contact information of the oncologist and the hospital where the patient is going to be treated

- Dental History
  - Last visit to the dentist and type of treatment received
  - Current dental problems
  - Oral hygiene habits
  - Name of the dentist and contact information

- Clinical Pearls:
  - Check for drugs that induce xerostomia
  - Determine whether patients are going to get chemotherapy that may cause a decrease in blood counts which predispose to infection
  - Determine whether patients have low platelets as this may predispose to bleeding
  - Check to see if radiation will include the oral cavity

COMMUNICATION WITH THE ONCOLOGY TEAM

Collaboration with the oncology team is vital. This will facilitate access to medical information that may impact the provision of dental care. Increasingly, patients have multiple physicians involved in their care. In general, one physician will usually take charge of coordinating care. Patients can usually identify the coordinating physician and provide contact information. Dentists are advised to contact the coordinating physician directly. This will allow a mutual exchange of information and treatment recommendations. It is particularly important to inform the oncology team of any oral health issues that may predispose to treatment related toxicities.

For patients currently undergoing cancer treatment, any dental treatment recommendations should be discussed with the cancer management team prior to actual dental treatment. Patients being treated with chemotherapy will have various degrees of myelosuppression, rendering them at risk for infections and bleeding. In such cases, most elective, non-emergency dental treatment can be postponed until after the completion of the cancer treatment. For emergency dental treatment, hemostasis, prevention of infection, and medication interactions should be discussed with the medical team.

For patients who have had cancer treatment in the past, ongoing communication remains important. Although patients may have recovered from the acute side effects of therapy, late side effects may affect oral health. For example, it may be necessary to contact the Radiation Oncologist for information on radiation portals for head and neck cancer patients prior to dental extractions. Patients who have undergone bone marrow transplant may develop oral complications of chronic graft versus host disease. This type of information is more reliable when received directly from the medical team than from the patient. Often patients are unsure of treatment details and the current status of their disease. While some patients are well informed, they are by far the exception and not the rule.

CANCER STAGING AND PROGNOSIS

Numerous staging systems have been created to guide treatment and allow prediction of prognosis for various cancers. In the United States, most tumors are staged using the the American Joint Committee /Union Internationale Contre le Cancer (AJCC/UICC) TNM classification system. The TNM system provides descriptors for the extent of the primary cancer (T-stage), nodal involvement (N-stage) and metastases (M-stage). The data is combined into a table with overall stage. Distinct staging systems exist for specific sites and/or histologic subtypes, thus the system is extensive, exact and complicated. Despite decades of development, the TNM system is not an effective staging system for all cancers. For example, the TNM staging does not work well for gliomas which rarely spread to lymph nodes or metastatic sites. Patients with lymphoid malignancies are classified based on the World Health Organization Classification of Lymphoid Neoplasms. Information regarding staging for all malignancies can be found in the AJCC Cancer Staging Handbook which is available on line.

It is not critical for oral health care providers to understand the nuances of cancer staging. What is important is to understand the short and long term prognosis for the patients undergoing dental therapy. This information can be best obtained from members of the Oncology team.

Patients may be reluctant to discuss long term prognosis, particularly if survival is expected to be short. Understanding prognosis facilitates the decision making process used to decide whether to provide radical, conservative, or palliative dental care based on the stage of cancer the patient has and the expected prognosis.

There are a number of critical questions regarding prognosis which should be directed to the Oncology team. First, is the cancer being treated with curative intent? If so, what is the chance for cure? If the tumor is not curable, what is the likely overall survival? If survival is brief, reasonable palliative options for severe dental problems should be discussed with the Oncology team. It is also important to know what the patient has been told and what they understand so that discussions can be appropriately directed.

TREATMENT AND SUPPORTIVE SERVICES IN THE MANAGEMENT OF CANCER

TREATMENT STRATEGIES

Surgery

Dating back a millennium, surgery is the oldest method for treating cancer. Oncologic surgeons are a growing group of specialists who provide care to cancer patients within their surgical specialty. Oncologic surgeons play a critical role in the management of cancer patients throughout the trajectory of their disease process, and should be considered an integral part of the treatment team. First, surgical procedures may be necessary to obtain tissue for histological diagnosis. Second, surgical assessment may be needed to determine the extent of disease. For example, head and neck cancer patients frequently undergo direct laryngoscopy to help stage their cancer. In addition, surgical resection is used with curative intent and for a number of tumors it remains the cornerstone of treatment. Surgeons also may aid in supportive care by placement of access devices such as portacaths or peritoneal catheters for chemotherapy administration. They may also perform procedures that are aimed at palliation. For example, patients with bowel obstruction may require surgical intervention for relief of symptoms. Finally, surgeons may perform surgical procedures aimed at reconstruction or rehabilitation of deficits secondary to cancer and its therapy.

Radiation Therapy

Radiation therapy is the therapeutic use of ionizing radiation to destroy cancer cells. Ionizing radiation kills primarily by damage to cellular DNA. This usually leads to cell death within several divisions. The changes that result in cell death occur in both normal tissue and the tumor. The ability of ionizing radiation to destroy a tumor without unacceptable damage to normal tissue is due to the biological differences between the two. Tumor cells are less able to repair the damage from the radiation because of genetic alterations, decreased vascularity, and hypoxia. Repopulation of cells occurs after radiation for both normal and tumor cells. Normal cells are able to respond with more rapid cell proliferation than tumor cells.

Radiation may be administered using two general techniques: brachytherapy and external beam (teletherapy). Brachytherapy places the radiation source in close proximity to the target volume. For example, implanted radioactive seeds are a commonly used technique for the treatment of prostate cancer. With external beam, the radiation source is at a distance from the patient. The vast majority of patients who receive radiation therapy are treated with external beam.

Similar to surgery, radiation therapy is a local treatment. It can be used with curative intent in localized tumors. The selection of patients for radiation therapy versus surgery is based on the size of the tumor, radiosensitivity and radiocurability, and the function or cosmetic results when compared to surgery. If an early laryngeal cancer can be treated with radiation therapy without affecting vocal quality, radiation may be chosen over surgical excision. On the other hand, small tumors of the lung may be hard to target with radiation due to respiratory interference, thus surgery is the preferred treatment modality. In addition to curative intent therapy, radiation plays a critical role in palliation for patients with disseminated disease. For example, patients with painful bone metastases may receive palliative radiation with the anticipation of good symptom control.

Radiation treatment planning is complex and requires the assistance of physicists well versed and experienced in radiation treatment planning. During radiation treatment planning, the following parameters will be determined:

- the goal of therapy (cure or palliation)
- the total dose of radiation required to attain that goal (in Gray or centiGray, Gy, cGy)
- the daily radiation dose (fraction size)
- the size of the radiation field (port size)

Some tumors are very radiation sensitive and respond to moderate doses of radiation therapy. For other tumors, higher doses of radiation are required for cure. In these instances, the ability to deliver higher doses of radiation to the tumor has been limited by normal tissue damage. Advances in radiation techniques have allowed the radiation to be delivered selectively to the tumor while avoiding critical normal structures. One such technique that is commonly used is intensity-modulated radiation therapy (IMRT). IMRT is standard for patients with head and neck cancer where avoiding high doses of radiation to the salivary glands has been demonstrated to decrease late effect xerostomia.

Systemic Therapy

Over the past fifty years, a large number of pharmacological agents have been developed that are either tumorstatic or tumoricidal. These systemic agents may be given with the following intent:

- Cure (such as leukemia or lymphoma)
- As a part of a combined modality treatment regimen to enhance outcomes (such as combined chemoradiation for head and neck cancers)
- As adjuvant therapy after surgery to prevent recurrence (as in stage III colon cancer)
- To improve survival in patients with non-curable disease
- For palliation of symptoms.

It is critical to know the goal of therapy in order to help make decisions regarding the balance between treatment efficacy and toxicity. In patients for whom cure is possible, severe chemotherapy-related side effects are usually deemed acceptable. In patients for whom treatment is purely palliative, side effects should be kept to a minimum.

The mechanism of action of systemic agents varies widely from alkylating agents that damage DNA to targeted agents that block specific biological pathways. As would be expected, the toxicities that result also vary dramatically from drug to drug. In general, when agents are given in combination, the toxicity is expected to increase. High dose chemotherapy with stem cell rescue is used in highly selective malignancies where curative doses of chemotherapy cause ablation of the bone marrow.

It is not expected that oral health providers would know the toxicities for the ever-changing and ever-expanding armamentarium of systemic agents used for the treatment of cancer. By communicating with the treating Oncologist, one can be apprised of the drugs being used, the treatment schedule, and any anticipated complications that may impact oral care or dental procedures. Complications of cancer treatment are typically divided into acute (or early) and chronic (or late). Some of the toxicities relevant to oral health providers are listed in Table 2.

Table 2
Common Toxicities Associated with Systemic Cancer Treatment

Mucositis	A pan-tissue inflammation that manifests with erythema and ulceration of the lining of the gastrointestinal system. The manifestation of mucositis depends on the site within the alimentary canal that is affected. When present in the oral cavity, mucositis results in pain and ulceration, decreased oral intake, decreased oral hygiene and altered speaking ability.
Thrombocytopenia	Most common in patients treated with high doses of chemotherapy or those with hematologic disorders. Severe bleeding generally does not develop until the platelet count is below 10,000 to 20,000/mm^3. That being said, elective procedures such as dental extraction are usually delayed unless the platelet count is above 30,000/mm^3. If a dental procedure is urgent and a patient has severe thrombocytopenia, platelet transfusion may be undertaken prior to the procedures. Coordination of medical and dental intervention is of utmost importance for a positive outcome.
Neutropenia	Neutrophils are critical for fighting infection. The risk of infection is related to the neutrophil count: the lower the count, the higher the risk for infection. Patients with mild or moderate neutropenia generally are able to mount an adequate response to infections. However, patients with severe neutropenia (<500 cells/microL) are susceptible to potentially life threatening infections.
Taste alterations	Although less frequent and severe than radiation induced taste alterations, chemotherapy induced taste changes may cause decreased oral intake, decreased appetite, nausea and gagging.
Xerostomia	Symptoms are less severe than radiation induced xerostomia and tend to be transient. That being said, chemotherapy induced xerostomia may result in discomfort, altered food intake, decreased taste and increased risk for decay and infection.

Combination Therapy

Medical research continues to combine treatment modalities to optimize treatment outcome. The major factors to be considered in the determination of the appropriate treatment are:

1. Rate of cure for each combined modality versus single modality therapy
2. Relative morbidity of combined modality versus single modality therapy.
3. Function and aesthetic results of various treatment options.

In general, combined modality therapy is associated with substantial increase in acute toxicities (that usually occur during and immediately after the end of therapy) and late toxicities (that usually occur after completion of therapy and can remain with the patient for years). Not all patients are able to tolerate aggressive combined modality treatment. Patients with significant co-morbidities may be best served by less aggressive treatment.

SUPPORTIVE SERVICES

Nutrition

Nutrition is a critical issue for all patients with cancer. Diet adequacy may be affected by a number of factors including:

- Nausea and vomiting due to chemotherapy or radiation therapy
- Cachexia secondary to systemic effects of cancer
- Decreased oral intake due to mucositis associated pain and swelling
- Decreased oral intake due to phlegm production from tumor or radiation
- Taste alterations
- Dental issues including infection, extraction, poor fitting dentures
- Pain secondary to osteonecrosis
- Alterations in swallowing function

Health care providers should obtain a weight loss history in patients with any of the issues listed above. A consultation with a certified dietician should be made if significant weight loss or significant alterations in dietary intake are noted.

Speech and Language Therapy

Patients with cancers or cancer therapy that affects the upper aerodigestive tract may have alterations in swallowing or speech function. Altered swallowing function may lead to decreased oral intake, aspiration, infection and chronic respiratory damage. Patients with impediments in speaking may experience social handicaps that result in job loss, social isolation and social phobia. Patients with identified issues in swallowing and speaking should be referred for evaluation by a certified Speech and Language Therapist.

Physical Therapy

Patients may experience alterations in range of motion in the neck, shoulders and jaw as a result of therapy for head and neck cancer. Trismus is a very common problem that can progress rapidly and limit oral intake and dental hygiene. This side effect of head and neck cancer surgery and radiation is often overlooked by the treating physicians. If trismus is identified, immediate referral to physical therapy is indicated. The use of mechanical devices to stretch the jaw may be useful in treating trismus or preventing further functional loss.

2 – Dental Considerations Prior to Cancer Treatment

The goal of treating a patient prior to the start of cancer therapy is to diagnose oral disease, establish oral health as quickly and effectively as possible, and establish an oral hygiene protocol. The decision about treating the patient with a radical protocol (extractions) or conservative protocol (caries control, restorative work) will depend on several factors including the staging of the cancer, the type of cancer therapy being proposed, oral hygiene habits of the patient, and time available prior to the start of therapy. This is also the time to provide patient counseling regarding what type of oral toxicities to expect to occur, oral health maintenance, proper nutrition, and when to contact the dentist in case oral complications develop.

Pre-treatment Visit

- Thorough clinical examination
  - Extraoral:
    - Observe any asymmetry, skin abnormalities or lesions
    - Palpate for abnormal lymph nodes, salivary glands, tenderness in muscles of mastication and TMJ
  - Intraoral:
    - Observe and palpate soft tissue for consistency, erythema, ulceration erosion, hemorrhage, swelling, or other lesions
      - Buccal mucosa
      - Labial mucosa
      - Alveolar mucosa
      - Palate and uvula
      - Oropharynx and pillars of fauces
      - Tongue
      - Floor of mouth and lingual of mandible
      - Nature and quantity of saliva
      - Have patient swallow
    - Periodontal assessment: probing depths, bleeding, plaque and calculus, acute infection or abscess
    - Dental caries and non-serviceable restorations
    - Removable prosthodontic appliances should be evaluated for fit. Tissue-borne appliances may exacerbate mucositis.

- Correlate radiographic examination
  - Panoramic image is usually acceptable, but if evaluating a patient for head and neck radiation or pre-IV bisphosphonate therapy, it is often necessary to add periapical and/or bitewing images
  - Rule out impacted teeth, retained root tips, latent osseous disease that could exacerbate during immunosuppressive cancer therapy

Treatment plan should include:

- Calculus removal, prophylaxis, fluoride treatment
- Oral hygiene instructions
- Diet counseling: encourage non-cariogenic diet
- Eliminate all sources of irritation or infection
    - Non-restorable teeth (poor or hopeless prognosis, acute infection, or severe periodontal disease) should be extracted.
    - Sharp, bony edges of alveolus should be trimmed and smoothed to facilitate healing.
    - Primary closure of surgical site should be obtained, with adequate time for healing before induction of cancer treatment.
- Symptomatic non-vital permanent teeth should receive root canal treatment at least one week before initiation of cancer treatment to allow sufficient time to assess treatment success before the initiation of treatment
- Temporary restorations can be placed and elective treatment (cosmetic, prosthodontic, asymptomatic endodontic) can be delayed

For children who will have chemotherapy:

- Mobile primary teeth and those expected to be exfoliated during chemotherapy should be extracted
- Gingival opercula should be evaluated for surgical removal to prevent entrapment of food debris
- Orthodontic bands should be removed before starting chemotherapy

GUIDELINES FOR TOOTH EXTRACTION IN PATIENTS SCHEDULED TO RECEIVE HEAD AND NECK RADIATION (INCLUDING THE MOUTH) OR CHEMOTHERAPY

Indicators of Extraction:

- Pocket depths 5 mm or greater, excessive mobility, purulence on probing
- Periapical inflammation present (and endodontic treatment not possible or not desired)
- A tooth is broken-down, non-restorable, non-functional or partially erupted and the patient is noncompliant with oral hygiene measures
- Patient has no interest in saving tooth/teeth
- Tooth is associated with an inflammatory (e.g., pericoronitis), infectious or malignant osseous disease

Dental Extraction Guidelines:

Radiation therapy: *

- Extraction performed with minimal trauma at least 2 weeks, (ideally at least 3 weeks) before initiation of radiation therapy.

Chemotherapy: *

- Extraction performed with minimal trauma at least 7 days, (ideally at least 2 weeks) before initiation of chemotherapy.
- Perform a conservative alveoloplasty by smoothing bone at wound margins to eliminate sharp edges
- Obtain primary closure
- Avoid intra-alveolar hemostatic packing agents that can serve as a nidus of microbial growth
- May need to transfuse if the platelet count is less than 20,000-30,000/mm^3
- Delay if the white blood count is less than 2,000/mm3 or the absolute neutrophil count is less than 500 - 1000/mm^3 or expected to be this level within 10 days; alternatively prophylactic antibiotics (e.g. penicillin or cephalosporin) can be used with extractions that are mandatory

**** In select circumstances when healing will not be compromised, a minimum of 10 days can be used. Alternatively, if these time recommendations cannot be met before initiation of chemotherapy, non-surgical root canal therapy can be performed to reduce the number of viable microbes, then the extraction can be performed after the white blood cell count returns to sufficient levels.***

Guidelines for Patients Who Will be Intubated During Surgery to Treat Malignancy

- Evaluate dentition for problems that can occur during intubation.
- Document the status of the teeth and appliances as a record of existing conditions.
    - May be necessary to resolve damage claims after surgery.
    - Radiographic records sufficient to view the entire oral cavity and dentition.
- Eliminate teeth that may become dislodged and present an aspiration risk during intubation.
- Remove gross calculus, loose restorations, crowns, and appliances that may become dislodged during intubation.
- Educate the patient on concerns and treatment recommendations.
- Document all accepted treatment and refused treatment recommendations.

3 – Dental Considerations During Cancer Treatment

Management of Dental Emergencies During Chemotherapy

Abscess of periodontal or endodontic origin:

- Consultation with the physician regarding status of immune system
- Transfuse if the platelet count is less than 20,000-30,000/mm^3
- Use perioperative antibiotics (e.g. penicillin) if the white blood count is less than 2,000/mm^3 or the absolute neutrophil count is less than 500 - 1000/mm^3
- Chemotherapy may need to be suspended so that infection can be managed

Extractions:

- It is best to treat dental infections with antibiotics when a chemotherapy-associated nadir (absolute neutrophil count < 500 mm^3) is present.
- Assure gentle tissue manipulation if an extraction is deemed necessary
- Concern for hemostasis: coagulation status (PT, PTT) and adequate platelet count (>30,000/mm^3)
- Suture as needed

Restorative needs:

- Smooth rough edges of broken fillings or teeth to protect soft tissue from injury
- Recement crowns only if retention is assured; aspiration of loose restorations may lead to pneumonia

Pain medication:

- Caution with the use of aspirin or other NSAIDS that may interfere with platelet function.

Oral Complications During Chemotherapy

- Nausea and vomiting (acute onset)
- Mucositis: starts about second week
- Oral pain
- Taste alteration: starts about second week
- Secondary infections (fungal, bacterial, viral)
- Bleeding
- Hypersensitive teeth (acute and delayed onset)

Complications of Head and Neck Radiotherapy

Early

- Nausea and vomiting (acute onset)
- Mucositis: starts about second week
- Taste alteration: starts about second week
- Xerostomia: starts about second week
- Secondary infections (fungal, bacterial, viral). Risk increases with xerostomia.

Late

- Radiation caries (delayed onset)
- Limited mouth opening- trismus (delayed onset)
- Osteoradionecrosis (delayed onset): more common in mandible than in maxilla
- Pulpal pain and necrosis (delayed onset)

Oral Complications During Hematopoietic Stem Cell Transplant (HSCT) Therapy

1. Preconditioning stage (due to the disease itself)

- Oral infections: dental caries, endodontic infections, periodontal disease (gingivitis,periodontitis), mucosal infections (i.e., viral, fungal, bacterial)
- Gingival leukemic infiltrates
- Metastatic cancer
- Oral bleeding due to thrombocytopenia
- Oral ulceration

2. Conditioning stage (pancytopenia)

- Oropharyngeal mucositis
- Oral infections: mucosal infections (i.e., viral, fungal, bacterial), periodontal infections
- Hemorrhage
- Xerostomia
- Taste dysfunction
- Neurotoxicity: dental pain, muscle tremor (e.g., jaws, tongue)

3. Engraftment stage:

- Oral infections: mucosal infections (i.e., viral, fungal, bacterial)
- Acute graft-versus-host-disease (GVHD)—first 100 days
- Xerostomia
- Hemorrhage
- Neurotoxicity: dental pain, muscle tremor (e.g., jaws, tongue)
- Granulomas/papillomas (HPV)

4. Immune Reconstitution (some acute complications continue at this stage; others are chronic)

- Oral infections: mucosal infections (i.e., viral, fungal, bacterial)
- Chronic GVHD
- Dental/skeletal growth and development alterations (pediatric patients)
- Xerostomia
- Relapse-related oral lesions
- Second malignancies

5. Maintenance or Long-term Survival (Chronic or late complications – see section 4)

- Relapse or second malignancies
- Dental/skeletal growth and development alterations

4 – Dental Considerations Post Cancer Treatment

Routine Dental Care

After cancer therapy ends, the provision of dental care and oral health maintenance will depend on the type of therapy the patient was treated with and the observed recovery.

Patients treated with chemotherapy

Chemotherapy agents can cause severe suppression of the bone marrow resulting in low blood cell counts. Patients with low blood cell counts are at increased risk for anemia, infections and bleeding. Therefore, recovery of cell counts to normal levels is imperative before any dental treatment can be done. The Oral Health Professional should obtain information on patient's blood cell counts and if any medication that can cause complications is still being used (e.g., corticosteroids). The oncology team can assure when dental care provision will be safe. In some instances, several cycles of chemotherapy are used to treat cancer. Routine dental care is usually avoided until the end of all the cycles. In case of dental emergencies, treatment must be coordinated with the oncologist.

Patients treated with HSCT or bone marrow transplants received high-dose chemotherapy and are maintained on immunosuppressive therapy until the risk of rejection decreases. Some may have chronic graft-versus-host disease that can appear as oral ulcerations that are uncomfortable as well as a potential for infection. For many HSCT patients, elective care may need to be delayed until the immune system has stabilized (e.g, normal blood counts). Emergency care should be provided as needed to assure comfort as well as reduce the potential for systemic infection. Therefore, it is recommended that before any dental intervention in these patients, a consultation with the oncology team is secured for determination of health status, immunosuppression and risk for complications.

Patients treated with radiation therapy of the head and neck

Radiation therapy (RT) of the head and neck area where portals include the oral cavity may alter the capacity of the oral tissues to regenerate and heal. In addition, RT involving oral cavity and salivary glands will cause severe mucositis in about 100% of the patients and depending on the dose, severe damage of major salivary glands. With decreased salivary secretion and painful ulcers, the patient will have difficulty swallowing, chewing and speaking. During this time, the most important oral care should aim to improving mucosal moistening and oral hygiene. Routine dental care will be delayed until the oral conditions improve. Because of thick saliva secretion, ulcerations and trismus, patients will have trouble opening the mouth making dental care impossible. Emergencies must be resolved on a case by case basis and in coordination with the radiation oncologist. Once the oral cavity improves, routine dental treatment can resume.

Patients who have been successfully treated for cancer should receive normal dental care. However, there is an increased risk for second primary cancers in these patients, especially in patients who have had HSCT. The dentist should be vigilant in completing a comprehensive head and neck exam as certain types of cancer are more likely to metastasize to the orofacial region, such as breast, kidney, lung, prostate, or thyroid, although this is rare. Restoring the patient's ability to eat assures that proper nutrition is possible. The patient's self-esteem also benefits from having a healthy, pain-free mouth and smile.

PATIENTS RECEIVING SUPPORTIVE THERAPY — BONE-MODIFYING AGENTS AND ANTIANGIOGENICS AND JAW OSTEONECROSIS ASSOCIATED WITH MEDICATIONS (JOM)

Some types of cancer may lead to painful and weakened bones. The bisphosphonate medications and denosumab are often used to treat and prevent skeletal morbidity associated with multiple myeloma or bone metastases from solid tumors.

Definition and Clinical Appearance of JOM

- Unexpected area of necrotic bone in the oral cavity that persists more than 8 weeks
- Previous or current use of one of the medications (see below)
- May be acutely painful when secondarily infected
- Soft tissue inflammation and infection
- Associated with tooth extraction or surgical manipulation of bone, although spontaneous symptoms may be misinterpreted and lead to surgery
- Radiographic: similar appearance to osteomyelitis

Common medications

1. Bisphosphonates
    a. Intravenous use, typically prescribed to patients with bone malignancies or metastases of other cancers to the bones
        i. zoledronate (Zometa®, Reclast® - marketed for osteoporosis as once yearly dosing)
        ii. pamidronate (Aredia®, may also be given to children with osteogenesis imperfecta)
    b. Oral (for treatment of osteoporosis, rarely for Paget's disease of bone)
        i. alendronate (Fosamax®)
        ii. risedronate (Actonel®, Atlevia™)
        iii. pamidronate (Aredia®)
        iv. ibandronate (Boniva®)

2. Denosumab: monoclonal antibody anti-RANKL (Xgeva™, Prolia®)
    a. Subcutaneous use, typically prescribed to patients with multiple myeloma and advanced cancers with bone metastasis, and patients with osteoporosis

3. Antiangiogenics
    a. Typically prescribed to patients with advanced cancers
        i. bevacizumab (Avastin®)

Treatment recommendations

Treatment can follow guidelines based on clinical staging of the lesions proposed by the American Academy of Oral and Maxillofacial Surgery (see Table 3) addressing bisphosphonate-related osteonecrosis of the jaw (BRONJ). In general, a conservative management of the lesions is recommended for lesions in stages 1 to 2 and a surgical approach with surgical resection for stage 3 lesions.

Table 3

Staging of Bisphosphonate-related Osteonecrosis of the Jaw*¶

At Risk	No apparent necrotic bone in patients who have been treated with either oral or intravenous bisphosphonates
Stage 0	No clinical evidence of necrotic bone, but non-specific clinical findings and symptoms
Stage 1	Exposed and necrotic bone in patients who are asymptomatic and have no evidence of infection
Stage 2	Exposed and necrotic bone associated with infection as evidenced by pain and erythema in the region of the exposed bone with or without purulent drainage
Stage 3	Exposed and necrotic bone in patients with pain, infection, and one or more of the following: exposed and necrotic bone extending beyond the region of alveolar bone (i.e., inferior border and ramus in the mandible, maxillary sinus and zygoma in the maxilla) resulting in pathologic fracture, extra-oral fistula, oral antral/oral nasal communication, or osteolysis extending to the inferior border of the mandible or sinus floor

** Exposed bone in the maxillofacial region without resolution in 8-12 weeks in persons treated with a bisphosphonate who have not received radiation therapy to the jaws.*

¶ Adapted from Ruggiero SL, et al. J Oral Maxillofac Surg 2009;67(Suppl 1):2-12.

Conservative protocol:

- smooth rough edges and remove bony sequestra that are readily removed
- systemic antibiotics when active infection with purulent exudate is present
    - IV antibiotics may be necessary for non-responders that present progression and the clinical lesion cannot be controlled with oral antibiotics
- chlorhexidine rinse 2-4 times/day
- pain medication if necessary
    - soft mouth guard to cover rough area, protecting adjacent tissue
- close follow-up for acute cases
- routine professional oral hygiene maintenance at short interval (3 months)

Surgical protocol:

- systemic antibiotics
- surgical resection of necrotic bone
- recovery of surgical bed with soft tissue
- bone graft placement when indicated
- oral hygiene maintenance and chlorhexidine rinse 2-4 times/day
- close follow up to document healing

5 – Oral Complications and Treatment

Early or Acute Complications

Oral Mucositis (Stomatitis)

Pathogenesis:

- Oral mucositis describes inflammation of oral mucosa resulting from cytotoxic chemotherapeutic agents used primarily to treat the malignancy. The epithelial cells lining the pharynx, esophagus and the rest of the gastrointestinal tract may also be involved. Rapidly dividing cells are the most likely to be affected.
- Mucositis is exacerbated by salivary dysfunction, oral candidosis, and malnutrition.
- The severity of mucositis is closely related to the degree of neutropenia that is caused by the chemotherapy. The most severe cases of mucositis are seen with the treatment of leukemia in which the patient receives hematopoietic stem cell transplant. Chemotherapy to treat breast cancer and other solid organ tumors may also result in varying degrees of mucositis.
- Mucosal breakdown is drug and dose dependent and typically occurs 7 to 10 days following initiation of therapy.
- Mucositis is self-limited when uncomplicated by infection and typically heals within 2 to 4 weeks after cessation of cytotoxic chemotherapy.

Signs and Symptoms:

- Diffuse erythema on all mucosal surfaces, followed by epithelial erosion and ulceration
- Sometimes accompanied by edema
- Mild soreness to severe pain that can be characterized by the patient's ability to eat solid foods or need of liquid nutrition supplementation.
- Several assessment scales have been developed to measure the severity and therefore the treatment of mucositis The World Health Organization Oral Toxicity Scale uses anatomical, symptomatic, and functional components as follows:
    - Grade 0 = no oral mucositis
    - Grade 1 = soreness with or without erythema
    - Grade 2 = erythema, ulcers, and patient can swallow solid food
    - Grade 3 = ulcers with extensive erythema and patient cannot swallow solid food
    - Grade 4 = mucositis to the extent that alimentation is not possible

Differential Diagnosis:

- Oral candidosis
- Recurrent herpetic stomatitis
- Erythema multiforme
- Chemical or thermal burn

Management:

- Topical anesthetic agents

Ice chips: Allow ice to melt in mouth and swallow.

Rx: Viscous lidocaine HCl 2%.
Disp: 250 mL.
Sig: Swish and spit 5 mL for 5 minutes qid for pain.

Rx: Diphenhydramine (Children's Benadryl®) elixir 12.5 mg/5 mL (OTC).
Disp: 250 mL.
Sig: Swish and spit 5 mL qid for 5 minutes.

Note: Lidocaine or diphenhydramine can be mixed 1:1 with either kaolin & pectin (Kaopectate®), aluminum hydroxide & magnesium hydroxide (Maalox®), or sucralfate to increase mucosal binding.

- Mucosal coating agents such as methylcellulose (Zilactin®), cyanoacrylate, sucralfate
- Systemic analgesics as needed (see below).
- Saliva substitutes or stimulants (see below).
- Anti-infectives as indicated.
- Oral hygiene instructions including extra-soft toothbrush and avoid alcohol-based mouthwash.

Rx: Add 1⁄4 teaspoon baking soda and 1⁄8 teaspoon salt to 1 cup water.
Disp: 1 cup.
Sig: Rinse several times a day, especially after meals.

- Liquid nutritional supplements: Ensure®, Sustacal™
- For patients with hematologic malignancies, keratinocyte growth factor may decrease the incidence and duration of severe oral mucositis.

PAIN

Pathogenasis:

- Usually secondary to mucositis and/or infection
- May also be due to neurotoxicity of chemotherapeutic agents

Signs and Symptoms:

- Mucositis (see above)
- Pain may be acute, chronic, or intermittent, and related to treatment
- Pain may be so severe that patient is unable to eat, drink, swallow, or speak
- Affects mood and behavior
- May be so severe that therapy is interrupted

Differential Diagnosis:

- Dental or periodontal abscess
- Vesiculobullous disease (pemphigus, pemphigoid, etc.)
- Neurogenic pain
- Burning mouth syndrome
- Pain due to cancer itself
- Referred pain

Managment:

- Topical anesthetics (see above)
- Systemic analgesics should be prescribed with consideration to proper dosing and interactions to other medications that the patient is taking. Patients may be taking pain medication for non-dental pain and won't need additional prescriptions, *however,* do *not under-treat.*

> **Rx:** Ibuprofen 800mg.
> Disp: 30 tabs.
> Sig: Take 1 tab po q8h.

Non-steroidal anti-inflammatory drugs (NSAIDs) are useful in the treatment of mild to moderate pain. When inflammation is present, as with post surgical periods, the NSAID will also help treat the inflammation. NSAIDs also have antipyretic effects, and do not produce any physical or psychological dependence.

> **Rx:** Tylenol® #3 (others include Vicodin®, Lortab®, Percocet®).
> Disp: 28 tabs.
> Sig: Take 1-2 tabs po q4h prn pain.

Opioid analgesics should be added when the patient's pain is not managed by non-opioids alone. For patients who are non-ambulatory, intravenous opioids may be used by bolus, infusion, or patient controlled analgesia (PCA) pump. For chronic pain, transdermal delivery of fentanyl can be accomplished using a patch. Fentanyl citrate is also available for oral transmucosal absorption as a sweetened lozenge on a handle (Actiq®). This last analgesic does not work as a topical agent but is absorbed through the mucosa of the mouth and gastrointestinal tract, and is usually reserved for cancer related breakthrough pain in a patient who is already taking a strong opioid analgesic. In some patients, the side effects of opioids must be addressed: nausea and vomiting, constipation, iching, respiratory depression, and sedation.

For some patients, the use of other medications is part of the therapy of cancer pain. When there is pain of neuropathic origin, which includes pain from surgical trauma, radiation or chemo therapy, or tumor infiltration of the nerves, the addition of a coanalgesic may help. These medications include tricyclic antidepressants, anti-seizure medications (an off-label use), local anesthetic injections or patches, other topical medications such as capsaicin. See Burning Mouth Syndrome section.

Further consideration of post operative sequelae (e.g. scars from surgery or radiation) may indicate the need for muscle relaxants or systemic steroids. The use of anti-anxiety medications should be evaluated, and if appropriate, consultation with the patient's physician may be necessary.

Principles of Pain Management
Individualize the choice of pain medication, including route, dosage, and schedule
Use a regular schedule of dosing if pain is present most of the day, with a preference for a long duration
Know alternative medications, and rotate if tolerance develops
Follow the patient closely for adequate pain control and compliance
Recognize and treat side effects
Anticipate physical dependence and prevent withdrawal
Be aware of the psychological state of the patient

HEMORRHAGE

Pathogenesis:

- Chemotherapy that eliminated the bone marrow and production of platelets.
- Liver toxicity of chemotherapy that interferes with production of clotting factors.
- Mucositis leads to eroded blood vessels.

Signs and Symptoms:

- Spontaneous nose bleeds.
- Minor traumatic injuries continue to expand (purpura) or ooze (lacerations, erosions).
- Pallor due to occult bleeds.

Differential Diagnosis:

- Blood dyscrasias.
- Acquired coagulopathy or thrombocytopathy.
- Pancytopenia.

Management:

- Complete blood count with differential; platelets should be >30,000/mm^3.
- Check PT and PTT secondary to liver toxicity or disease.
- Transfusion of blood products before any surgical/dental treatment.
- Avoid NSAIDs.

INFECTIONS

Bacterial Infections

Pathogenesis:

- Extension of dental caries into pulpal tissues or advanced periodontal disease. Typically caused by pathogens related to dental caries (streptococcal organisms) or periodontal disease.

Signs and Symptoms:

- Swelling of the tissues around a tooth, in either a lingual or a buccal direction
- Sometimes presenting as a fluctuant mass with or without a sinus tract leading to the source of the infection.
- Pain may be localized to a tooth.
- May be accompanied by regional lymphadenopathy and fever
- Patient should be examined carefully to determine if the infection is localized or has spread beyond the dental-alveolar complex. May spread to the orbit superiorly or into the deep spaces of the neck. Close inspection of the oral tissues is needed to ensure that there is no elevation of the tongue or asymmetry of the posterior pharyngeal structures.

Management:

- Endodontic treatment or extraction of the infected tooth
- Incision or drainage if swelling is fluctuant
- Refer to oral surgeon if extensive regional spread is evident
- Antibiotic therapy may be necessary. In most cases, antibiotics are prescribed without culture of the area.

> **Rx:** Penicillin VK, 500 mg.
> Disp: 40 tabs.
> Sig: Take 1 tab q6h until all are taken.

For penicillin allergic patients:

> **Rx:** Clindamycin, 150 mg.
> Disp: 56 tabs.
> Sig: Take 2 tabs q6h until all are taken. Contact the doctor if diarrhea develops.

Viral Infections

a. Herpes Simplex

Pathogenesis:

- A transmissible infection with herpes simplex virus, usually type I or, less commonly, type II.
- Primary herpetic gingivostomatitis is rare in the older patient, and typical lesions are usually of the recurrent type.

Signs and Symptoms:

- Clear vesicles develop intra- and extraorally and rupture within hours, forming shallow ulcers.
- Recurrent lesions typically occur on mucosa bound to bone and on the keratinized mucosa of the lips (herpes labialis). They can also occur on other mucosal surfaces in the immunocompromised patient (e.g., those undergoing chemotherapy).
- Virus may be stimulated to replicate by sun exposure, cold air, stress, or due to immunosuppression. Prodromal sensation (tingling, burning, itching) may herald the recurrence.

Differential Diagnosis:

- Traumatic lesion
- Primary and secondary syphilis
- Impetigo
- Aphthous ulcer

Management:

- Treatment is more effective if started in the prodromal stage or when lesions first appear.

> **Rx:** Acyclovir ointment 5%.
> Disp: 15 g tube.
> Sig: Apply to area q2h for 7 days beginning with prodromal symptoms.

> **Rx:** Valtrex® 500 mg.
> Disp: 8 tabs.
> Sig: Take 4 tab first sign of prodrome, then take 4 tabs 12 hours later.

Systemic antiviral drugs for immunocompromised patients:

> **Rx:** Acyclovir 200 mg.
> Disp: 80 caps.
> Sig: Take 2 tabs qid for 10 days.

> **Rx:** Valtrex® 500 mg.
> Disp: 40 tabs.
> Sig: Take 1 tab qid for 10 days.

b. Varicella Zoster (Herpes Zoster, Shingles)

Pathogenesis:

- Reactivation of latent herpes varicella-zoster virus present since an original infection (chickenpox).

- Precipitating factors include thermal, inflammatory, radiologic, or mechanical trauma and immunocompromising states, including cancer, lymphoma, and Hodgkin's disease.
- Occurs more commonly in the elderly.

Signs and Symptoms:

- Painful segmental eruption of small vesicles that rupture to form confluent ulcers.
- Vesicles appear on the skin and oral mucous membranes and occur unilaterally along the ophthalmic, maxillary, or mandibular divisions of the trigeminal nerve.
- Ophthalmic division involvement requires close monitoring by an ophthalmologist.
- Postherpetic neuralgia can last for months following eruption of vesicles.

Differential Diagnosis:

- Herpes simplex.
- Erythema multiforme.

Management:

Rx: Valtrex 500 mg.
Disp: 80 tabs.
Sig: Take 2 tabs qid for □10 days.

Rx: Famciclovir 500 mg.
Disp: 21 tabs.
Sig: Take 1 tab tid for □7 days.

Rx: Acyclovir 200 mg.
Disp: 160 caps.
Sig: Take 4 caps qid for □10 days.

Systemic steroids may be used to treat severe postherpetic neuralgia and severe cases of zoster infection. Consultation with the patient's physician is recommended, especially in patients taking multiple medications or those who are immunosuppressed.

Rx: Prednisone 5 mg tabs.
Disp: 86 tabs.
Sig: Take 12 tabs qd for □2 days, 10 tabs qd for 2 days, 8 tabs qd for □2 days, 6 tabs qd for □2 days, 4 tabs qd for 2 days, 2 tabs qd for 2 days, 1 tab qd for 2 days. Consider therapy every other day to decrease immunosuppression.

NOTE: For the older patient with diabetes, osteoporosis, uncontrolled cardiovascular diseases, narrow-angle glaucoma, depression, or any other immunocompromising condition, consult with the patient's physician before initiating prednisone therapy. Side effects have occurred more commonly in long-term followup of patients taking systemic steroids versus topical steroids, whereas the percentage of patients responding to long-term therapy was the same.

Tricyclic antidepressants may be indicated for postherpetic neuralgia pain.

Fungal Infections (may occur in multiple forms: pseudomembranous, erythematous, hyperplastic, angular cheilitis)

Pathogenesis:

- The most common fungal organism isolated from the oral cavity is *Candida albicans*.
- Risk factors include salivary gland hypofunction; systemic treatment with antibiotics, corticosteroids, immunosuppressants, and cytotoxic agents; and diabetes mellitus and other immunocompromising conditions.
- Diagnosis requires positive culture, positive smear, or biopsy.

a. Pseudomembranous Candidosis (Thrush)

Signs and Symptoms:

- White slightly elevated plaques that can be wiped away leaving an erythematous area or pinpoint bleeds
- Patient may report burning or itching, as well as a lousy or metallic taste
- Direct smear can be fixed and stained using potassium hydroxide or periodic acid–Schiff reagent to reveal the *Candida* hyphae microscopically.
- In severely debilitated patients, extension of candidosis into the esophagus and trachea may prove fatal

Differential Diagnosis:

- Radiation- or chemotherapy-induced mucositis
- Chemical or thermal trauma

b. Erythematous Candidosis (1- Denture sore mouth, 2- Median rhomboid glodssitis)

Signs and Symptoms:

- For patients with a removable appliance:
    - Mucosa beneath the denture is erythematous with a well-demarcated border
    - Patient may report keeping denture in mouth continuously (while sleeping)
    - Swabs from the mucosal surface may provide a prolific growth, but biopsy shows few *Candida* hyphae in spite of high serum and saliva antibodies to *Candida*
    - Treatment should include the denture.
- When tongue is involved, with or without appliance:
    - Depapillated erythematous area limited to median area of tongue with corresponding erythema on palate "kissing lesion"

Differential Diagnosis:

- Erosive lichen planus
- Mucositis
- Chemical or thermal trauma

c. Hyperplastic Candidosis (Cadidal Leukoplakia)

Signs and Symptoms:

- Confluent leukoplakic plaques that cannot be removed by wiping or scraping
- Biopsy reveals *Candida* invasion of oral epithelium
- Often lesions are asymptomatic

Differential Diagnosis:

- Leukoplakia
- Dysplasia
- Carcinoma in situ
- Squamous cell carcinoma
- Lichen planus
- Proliferative verrucous leukoplakia

Management fungal infections:

For superficial infections, the patient should be instructed to clean the oral cavity using irrigation and mechanical plaque removal before using the following topical agents:

Rx: Nystatin oral suspension 100,000 U/mL.
Disp: 60 mL.
Sig: Swish and swallow 5 mL qid for 5 minutes. Retain suspension in the mouth as long as possible. Contains sugar.

Rx: Nystatin troche 200,000 U.
Disp: 70 pastilles.
Sig: Let 1 pastille dissolve in mouth 5 times / day. Do not chew or swallow whole.

Rx: Nystatin 100,000 unit/gram cream or ointment.
Disp: 15 g tube.
Sig: Apply thin coat to affected areas after each meal and qhs.

Rx: Clotrimazole troches 10 mg.
Disp: 70 troches.
Sig: Let 1 troche dissolve in mouth 5 times / day. Do not chew or swallow whole.
Contains sugar

Rx for Dontures: Improve oral hygiene of the appliance, keep the denture out of the mouth for extended periods and while sleeping, soak for 30 minutes in solutions containing benzoic acid, 0.12% chlorhexidine, or 1% sodium hypochlorite, and thoroughly rinse. Apply a few drops of nystatin oral suspension or a thin film of nystatin ointment to the inner surface of the denture after each meal.

Persistent or locally invasive with or without systemic infections should be treated with systemic agents:

Rx: Ketoconazole 200 mg.
Disp: 20 tabs.
Sig: Take 1 tab daily for 10–14 days.

Rx: Fluconazole 100 mg. Disp: 20 tabs. Sig: Take 2 tabs stat and then 1 tab daily for 10–14 days.

Rx: Itraconazole 100 mg. Disp: 20 capsules. Sig: Take 1 tab bid for 10–14 days. Take capsules with food.

Rx: Amphotericin B (parenteral) use should be managed with the medical team.

d. Angular Cheilitis

Pathogenesis:

- Candidosis.
- Diminished occlusal vertical dimension.
- Vitamin B or iron deficiency.

Signs and Symptoms:

- Wrinkled and sagging skin at the lip commissures with desiccation.
- Mucosal cracking.
- Pain is usually related to manipulation of area with opening, chewing, speaking.

Differential Diagnosis:

- Actinic damage (sunburn).
- Dry chapped lips.
- Labial herpes simplex virus.
- Basal cell carcinoma.
- Squamous cell carcinoma.

Management: Repair vertical dimension if possible.

Rx: Nystatin 100,000 unit/gram ointment. Disp: 15 g tube. Sig: Apply to affected area after each meal and qhs. Concomitant intraoral antifungal treatment may be indicated (see the previous section).

If no resolution, consider that the area may also be infected with bacteria and treat with topical antibacterial ointment (available without a prescription) that can be alternated with antifungal and/or mixed together.

Late or Chronic Complications

XEROSTOMIA / SALIVARY GLAND FIBROSIS, SALIVARY HYPOFUNCTION (DRY MOUTH)

Pathogenesis:

- Multiple medications (anticholinergics, antihypertensives, antihistamines, psychotropics, antidepressants, antiparkinsonism agents).
- Head and neck radiation therapy.
- Sjögren's syndrome.
- Autonomic nerve dysfunction.
- Dehydration

Signs and Symptoms:

- Oral mucosa appears dry, pale, or atrophic.
- The tongue may be devoid of papillae with a fissured and inflamed appearance.
- Salivary gland obstructions owing to medication- and disease induced hypofunction lead to unilateral or bilateral glandular enlargement, frequently during mealtime.
- New and recurrent dental caries.
- Difficulty with speaking, chewing, swallowing, and tasting may occur.
- Fungal infections are common.

Management:

FOR DRUG-INDUCED DYSFUNCTION

- Consult with the physician to decrease drug dose, alter drug dosages, or substitute one xerostomic medication for a similar acting drug with fewer salivary side effects. The physician may be hesistant to changes medications especially if the patient has been stabilized for a chronic labile systemic condition.

SALIVARY SUBSTITUTES

- Sodium carboxymethyl cellulose 0.5% aqueous solution (OTC).
- Dispense 8 fl oz.
- Use as a rinse as frequently as needed.
- Commercial salivary substitutes (OTC) include Sage Moist-Plus® spray, Salivart®, MoiStir®, or Optimoist®.
- Commercial oral moisturizing gels (OTC) include Sage Moist-Plus Mouth Moisturizer® and Oral Balance®.

SYMPTOMATIC TREATMENTS

- Sip water frequently all day long.
- Let ice melt in the mouth.
- Restrict caffeine intake.
- Avoid mouth rinses containing alcohol.
- Humidify the sleeping area.
- Coat the lips with lubricant, such as Aquaphor®.

SALIVARY STIMULANTS

- Sugarless candies, sugarless mints, and sugarless gums can stimulate saliva from the remaining salivary tissue and may be the most appropriate method of controlling medication-induced salivary hypofunction.

- Two pharmaceutical agents (cholinergic agonists) can stimulate the remaining functional salivary tissue but will have limited success in patients who cannot produce saliva (such as after significant head and neck radiation for cancer). Patients can take these medications less frequently every day because they are primarily for patient comfort.

> **Rx:** Pilocarpine HCl 5 mg.
> Disp: 200 tabs.
> Sig: Take 1-2 tabs 30 minutes before meals. Maximum dose 6 tabs / day.

> **Rx:** Cevimeline HCl 30 mg.
> Disp: 60 tabs.
> Sig: Take 1 tablet tid. Dose may be raised to 45 mg tid.

Note:

May need 2–3 months to determine effectiveness. Side effects include sweating, chills, diarrhea, and increased need to urinate. May cause decreased vision capacity in low light. Avoid in patients with narrow-angle glaucoma, severe asthma, and pulmonary diseases. Use carefully in patients taking antihypertensive medications. Also may interfere with the therapeutic actions of many drugs. Cevimeline has a longer half-life than pilocarpine; therefore, only three doses / day are needed.

Patients with salivary dysfunction are at risk of developing caries (see "Dental Caries") and oral fungal infections (see "Fungal infections"). Consult with the patient's physician prior to prescribing these drugs if the patient is taking multiple medications.

Taste Alteration / Dysgeusia

Pathogensis:

- Mucositis may cause local destruction of taste cells when the dorsal surface of the tongue is affected.
- Fibrotic changes due to graft-versus-host disease.
- Xerostomia limits the dissolution of the molecule to be tasted, reducing access to the taste bud.

Signs and Symptoms:

- Ulcerations or erosions of dorsal surface of tongue.
- GVHD changes on surface of tongue.
- Lack of saliva.
- Patient complaint of limited sense of taste.

Differential Diagnosis:

- Chemotherapy mucositis.
- Graft-versus-host disease.
- Drug-related xerostomia.
- Candidosis.
- Alteration of sense of smell.

Management:

- Treatment of contributing factors (mucositis, xerostomia, candidosis).
- Assure sense of smell is intact.
- In addition to addressing the taste alteration, the patient may not be interested in eating; proper nutrition must be maintained while the patient is recovering from the stress of the cancer treatment.

DENTAL CARIES

Pathogensis:

- Gram-positive bacteria (primarily mutans streptococci group and lactobacilli).
- Risk factors associated with higher rates of caries formation include gingival recession (leading to root caries), salivary hypofunction, use of xerostomic medications, a diet high in fermentable sugars, poor oral hygiene, and inability to perform oral hygiene.

Signs and Symptoms:

- Discolored (dark yellow to black) hard to soft lesions on coronal or root surfaces surrounded by decalcified enamel when located on coronal surfaces.
- Failure of margins or loss of existing restorations (may only be radiographic evidence).
- Fracture of tooth structure.
- Mild sensitivity to acute pain depending on vitality of tooth and/or depth of decay.

Differential Diagnosis:

- Calculus.
- Enamel, dentinal, and cemental staining.
- Cervical abrasion or erosion.

Management:

- When decay is present, it must be removed and replaced with restorative materials. Depending on the location and extent of decay, and especially for root surface caries, fluoride-containing restorative materials should be used.
- Oral hygiene must be excellent.
- For patients with salivary gland hypofunction, see section on salivary gland dysfunction and xerostomia.
- Frequent recall visits
- Fluoride applications.

  Non-Rx:

  - 225 ppm NaF rinse
  - 1,000–1,500 ppm dentifrice

  Rx:

  - 5,000 ppm NaF gel and dentifrice,
  - 9,000–12,000 ppm gels/foams (used in dental offices),
  - 22,600 NaF varnish (applied in dental offices)

CARIES PREVENTION FOR ALL PATIENTS

1. Provide oral hygiene instructions.
2. Provide dietary counseling to decrease the frequency of consumption of fermentable carbohydrates.
3. Apply fluoride to teeth (see fluoride products above). Fluoride is available in a variety of formulations and concentrations, and the selection depends on caries risk, the severity of the decay, and the skills or resources available to the patient.
4. Use a non-Rx (over-the-counter [OTC]) fluoride-containing dentifrice after each meal.
5. Use a non-Rx (OTC) fluoride-containing rinse between meals if the patient is unable to brush. Rinse with 10 mL after meals for 60 seconds and expectorate. Avoid swallowing and rinsing or eating for 30 minutes following rinse.
6. Chew xylitol gum for 5 minutes between meals or after a meal when unable to brush teeth. Use xylitol mints 3 to 4 times daily between meals.

CARIES PREVENTION FOR HIGH-RISK PATIENTS

1. Prescribe a high-concentration fluoride dentifrice. Rx: Neutral pH sodium fluoride gel 1% or neutral pH sodium fluoride gel 1.1% (5,000 ppm). Disp: 1 tube. Sig: Apply a thin ribbon to a toothbrush. Brush thoroughly twice daily for 2 minutes, especially at bedtime. After use, expectorate. For best results, do not eat, drink, or rinse for 30 minutes.
2. Construct a custom fluoride delivery tray. Instruct the patient to place 1 drop of neutral sodium fluoride gel 1.0 or 1.1% per tooth in the custom tray and apply for 5 minutes daily. Avoid rinsing or eating for 30 minutes following treatment.
3. Apply fluoride varnish to teeth every 6 months.
4. Rx: Chlorhexidine 0.12% oral rinse. Disp: 250 mL. Sig: Rinse 15 mL for 30 seconds and expectorate twice daily for 2 weeks.

GINGIVAL ENLARGEMENT

Pathogenesis:

- Many patients who receive HSCT will be placed on anti-rejection drugs, including cyclosporine.
- Long-term use of this medication has been associated with gingival enlargement, perhaps due to hyperplasia of the tissue, or due to excess extra-cellular matrix.

Signs and Symptoms:

- Enlarged, fibrous, gingival tissue that may be normal in color or erythematous.
- Pseudopockets can develop.
- In some patients, the teeth are completely covered by the gingival tissue.
- Oral hygiene is difficult which may exacerbate the condition.

Differential Diagnosis:

- Gingivitis.
- ANUG.
- Leukemic gingival infiltrates.
- Enlargement due to calcium channel blockers or phenytoin.

Management:

- Improve oral hygiene.
- Gingival surgery (gingivectomy and / or gingivoplasty) but regrowth is common.
- Have physician consider an alternative immunosuppressant medication.

GRAFT VERSUS HOST DISEASE (GVHD)

Pathogenesis:

- Transplanted immune cells attack the patient's tissues.
- Acute GVHD occurs within first 100 days after engraftment.
- Chronic GVHD may occur 70 days after engraftment (with or without acute GVHD) and continue.

Signs and Symptoms:

Acute

- Mucosal atrophy.
- Lichenoid hyperkeratotic plaques and striae.
- Painful erosions and ulcerations may be present and be similar to oral mucositis.

Chronic

- Mucosal atrophy with erythema.
- Ulcerations and erosions.
- Lichenoid lesions.
- Xerostomia.
- Fibrotic changes to connective tissue rarely leads to limited opening and difficulty providing dental care.

Differential Diagnosis:

- Lichen planus
- Lichenoid reactions
- Chronic candidosis
- Recurrent herpes infection

Management:

Patients should be advised that the condition is often chronic and may recur when therapy is stopped. The therapeutic objective is to control the disease by reducing inflammation, especially when painful. Oral candidosis may develop in patients chronically using topical steroids. Concomitant conditions must be managed as well (xerostomia, caries, infections, temporomandibular joint dysfunction).

TOPICAL STEROIDS AND IMMUNOSUPPRESSANTS

Rx: Dexamethasone elixir 0.5 mg/5 mL.
Disp: 250 mL.
Sig: Swish and spit 5 mL qid for 5 minutes

Rx Clobetasol propionate 0.05% gel.
Disp: 15 g tube.
Sig: Apply thin layer to affected regions tid.

Rx: Fluocinonide 0.05% gel.
Disp: 15 g tube.
Sig: Apply thin layer to affected regions tid.

Rx Tacrolimus 0.1% ointment.
Disp: 15 g tube.
Sig: Apply thin layer to affected regions tid.

INJECTABLE STEROIDS

Rx: Betamethasone sodium phosphate-betamethasone acetate 3 mg/mL (Celestone Soluspan®)
Disp: 5 mL.
Sig: 0.2 mL intralesional injection.

Rx: Dexamethasone sodium phosphate 4 mg/mL.
Disp: 5 mL.
Sig: 0.5 mg intralesional injection.

Note: Injectable steroids can be combined with short-lasting (e.g. lidocaine 2%) or longer-lasting (e.g. bupivacaine hydrochloride 0.5%) injectable anesthetics to provide pain relief.

OSTEORADIONECROSIS

Pathogenesis:

- Ionizing radiation to treat oral/head and neck cancer causes fibrosis and loss of function of cells in adjacent tissues
- Associated with radiation dosage >6000cGy

Signs and Symptoms:

- Typically in the mandible
- Bone does not heal after tooth extraction
- Purulent exudate may be present
- Pain may be acute, chronic, or intermittent
- Radiographic appearance is moth-eaten or radiolucent

Differential Diagnosis:

- Osteomyelitis
- Jaw osteonecrosis associated with medication

Management:

- Prevention is best – provide any surgical treatment before radiation therapy
- Systemic antibiotics and analgesics
- Chlorhexidine rinses
- Conservative surgical debridement
- Hyperbaric oxy gen therapy to induce angiogenesis

JAW OSTEONECROSIS ASSOCIATED WITH MEDICATION (JOM)

Pathogenesis:

- Occurs in patients who have used anti-osteoporosis agents (e.g., bisphosphonates)
- Secondary to bone manipulation
- May also occur spontaneously

Signs and Symptoms:

- Unexpected area of necrotic bone in the oral cavity that persists more than 8 weeks
- May be acutely painful when secondarily infected
- Soft tissue inflammation and infection
- Associated with tooth extraction or surgical manipulation of bone, although spontaneous symptoms may be misinterpreted and lead to surgery
- Radiographic: similar appearance to osteomyelitis

Differential Diagnosis:

- Osteomyelitis
- Osteoradionecrosis

Management:

Conservative protocol:

- Smooth rough edges and remove bony sequestra that are readily removed
- Systemic antibiotics when active infection with purulent exudate is present
- IV antibiotics may be necessary for non-responders that present progression and the clinical lesion cannot be controlled with oral antibiotics
- Chlorhexidine rinse 2-4 times/day
- Pain medication if necessary
- soft mouth guard to cover rough area, protecting adjacent tissue
- Close follow-up for acute cases
- Routine professional oral hygiene maintenance at short interval (3 months).

Surgical protocol:

- Systemic antibiotics
- Surgical resection of necrotic bone
- Recovery of surgical bed with soft tissue
- Bone graft placement when indicated
- Oral hygiene maintenance and chlorhexidine rinse 2-4 times/day
- Close follow up to document healing

APPENDIX – SAMPLE CLINICAL IMAGES

DENTAL CONSIDERATIONS PRIOR TO CANCER TREATMENT

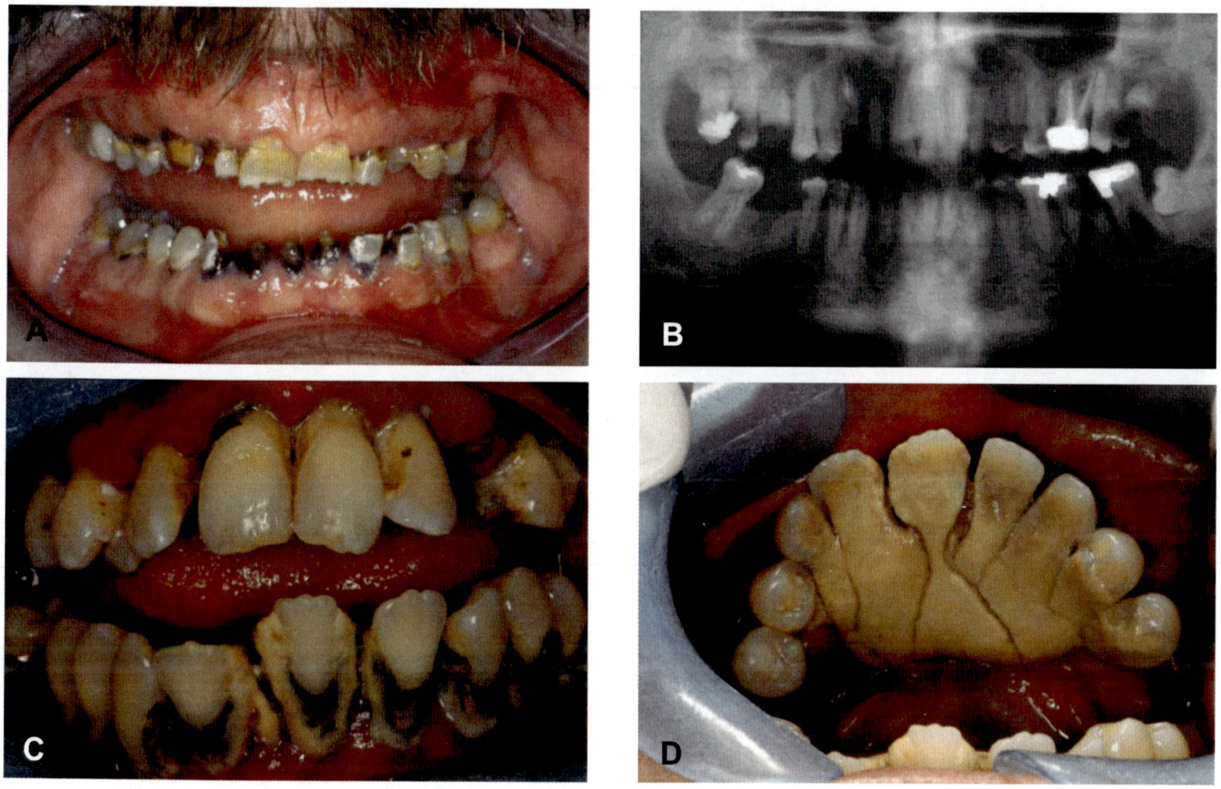

Figures A & B: Pre-therapy findings of rampant, hopeless caries. Treatment planned for full mouth extractions prior to radiation therapy to the head and neck.

Figures C & D: Pre-therapy findings of severe periodontitis with mobility; intubation risk. Treatment planned for full mouth extractions prior to radiation therapy to the head and neck.

DENTAL CONSIDERATIONS DURING CANCER TREATMENT

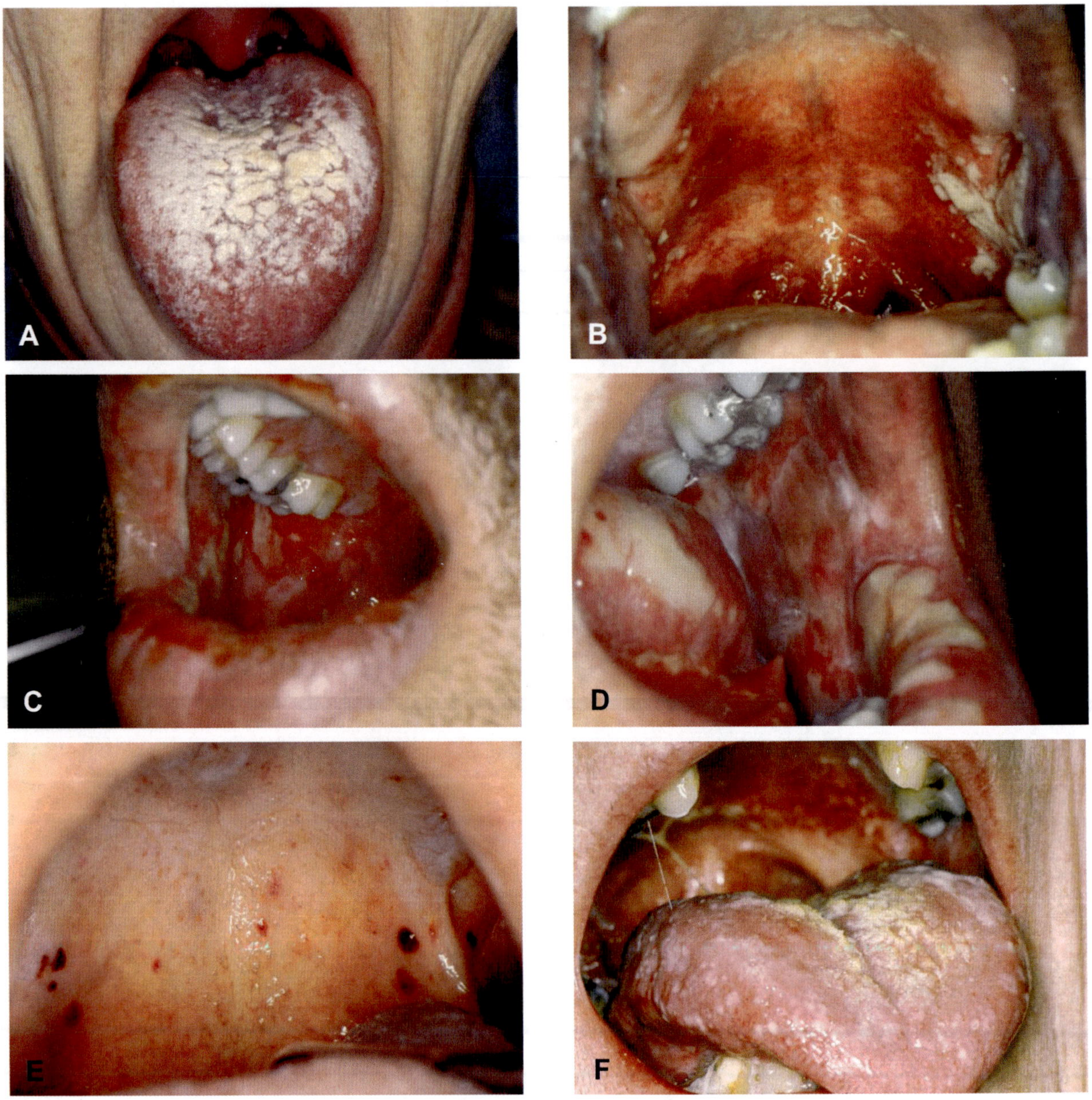

Figure A: Candidosis associated with chemotherapy; also note viscous saliva on uvula.

Figure B: Candidiosis associated with irradiation to the head and neck.

Figures C & D: Radiation-induced Grade 3 mucositis.

Figure E: Chmeotherapy-induced thrombocytopenia, note multiple petechiae.

Figure F: Chemotherapy-induced Grade 2 mucositis, candidosis, and xerostomia.

DENTAL CONSIDERATIONS POST CANCER TREATMENT

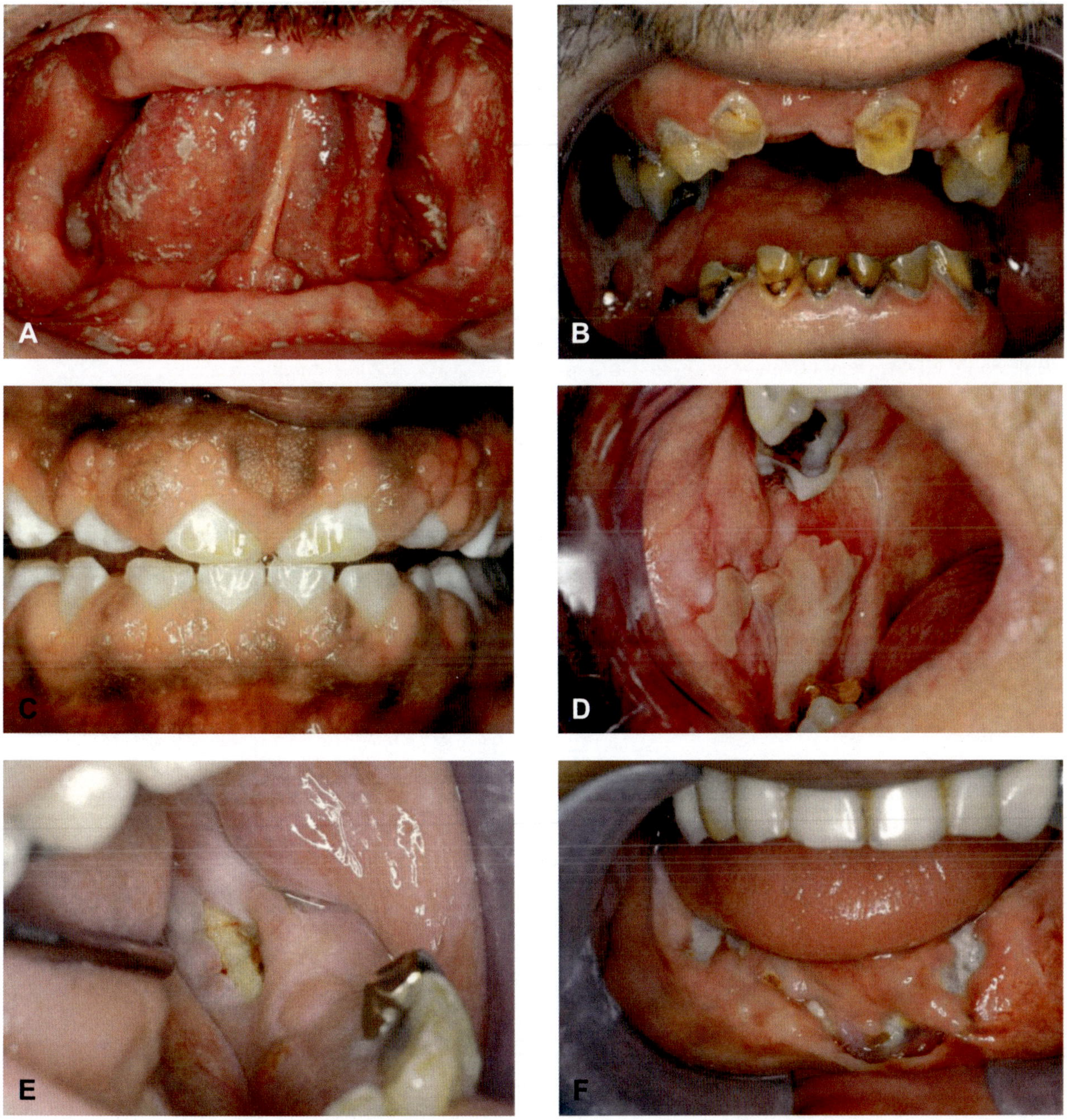

Figure A: Candidosis 2 year post radiation therapy in patient on multiple drying medications.

Figure B: Radiation caries; note viscous saliva indicative of xerostomia.

Figure C: Cyclosporine-induced gingival hyperplasia.

Figure D: Graft-versus-host-disease in bone marrow transplant patient.

Figures E & F: Jaw osteonecrosis associated with medication (JOM).

REFERENCES

Brennan MT, Woo SB, Lockhart PB. Dental treatment planning and management in the patient who has cancer. Dental Clinics of North America 2008; 52(1): 19-37.

Dental management of patients receiving oral bisphosphonate therapy: expert panel recommendations. J Am Dental Assoc 2006;137(8):1144-50.

Greenberg MS, Glick M. Burket's oral medicine, 11th ed. Hamilton, Ontario. BC Decker, 2008.

Keefe DM, Schubert MM, Elting LS, Sonis ST, Epstein JB, Raber-Durlacher JE, Migliorati CA, McGuire DB, Hutchins RD, Peterson DE. Updated clinical practice guidelines for the prevention and treatment of mucositis. *Cancer.* 2007;109(5):820-31.

Little, Falace, Miller, Rhodus. Dental Management of the Medically Compromised Patient, 7th ed. St. Louis, MO. Mosby. Ch. 26.

National Cancer Institute: PDQ® Oral Complications of Chemotherapy and Head/Neck Radiation. Bethesda, MD: National Cancer Institute. Date last modified 10/06/2009. Available at: http://cancer.gov/cancertopics/pdq/supportivecare/oralcomplications/HealthProfessional. Accessed 12/02/2010.

Ship JA. Oral health in geriatric patients, 2nd ed. Hamilton, Ontario. BC Decker, 2006.

Siegel MA, Silverman S Jr., Sollecito TP. Treatment of common oral conditions, 6th ed. Hamilton, Ontario. BC Decker, 2006.

Silverman S Jr, Eversole LR, Truelove EL. Essentials of oral medicine. Hamilton, Ontario. BC Decker 2001.

Sonis ST, Peterson DE, McGuire DB, eds. Mucosal injury in cancer patients: new strategies for research and treatment. J National Cancer Institute 2001;29:1-54.

SUGGESTED WEB SITES

Centers for Disease Control and Prevention: Fruits and Veggies Matter:
www.fruitsandveggiesmatter.gov/

American Academy of Oral Medicine:
www.aaom.com

Oral Cancer Foundation:
www.oralcancerfoundation.org

National Cancer Institute, Physician Data Query:
www.cancer.gov/cancertopics/pdq

National Cancer Institute, Surveillance Epidemiology and End Results Program:
http://seer.cancer.gov/

National Comprehensive Cancer Network Treatment Guidelines:
www.nccn.org/professionals/physician_gls/f_guidelines.asp

The American Academy of Oral Medicine
P.O. Box 2016
Edmonds, Washington 98020
Phone 425.778.6162 Fax 425.771.9588
www.aaom.com Email: Info@aaom.com

Application for Membership

Nominations must be returned as soon as possible to be acted upon at the next Academy meeting.

Eligibility for Membership

1. Nominee for **Regular Membership** shall be a graduate of an accredited Dental School or Medicine School and shall be a member of his/her representative National Society and shall pursue special interest or accomplishment in the field of Oral Medicine.

2. Nominee for **Affiliate Membership** (student) shall be a graduate of an accredited Dental or Medical School and shall be a member of his/her representative National Society and currently in training in a Postdoctoral program.

3. This application form should be **accompanied by a check (U.S. Funds) for $295.00 for Active Membership** or **$145.00 for Affiliate Membership (student)** which includes the one-time initiation fee. In event membership is not acted upon favorably, the total fee will be refunded. Make all checks payable to The American Academy of Oral Medicine, Inc. (Foreign checks must be made payable in U.S. Funds through a U.S. Bank.) The fiscal year for dues starts January 1.

4. After acceptance into the Academy, Active Membership dues are $295.00 annually and Affiliate Membership (student) dues are $145.00 annually, which shall include a subscription to ORAL SURGERY, ORAL MEDICINE, ORAL PATHOLOGY, ORAL RADIOLOGY, and ENDODONTOLOGY.

Dues are payable prior to election.

5. **Please attach a copy of your curriculum vitae or resume and a recent photo, for publication purposes, with this application.**

Applicant Name ______________________________ **Degree** ______________

Office Address ____

Telephone ____________________ Fax ____________________

Home Address ____

Telephone ____________________ Fax ____________________

Preferred Mailing address _______ Office _______ Home Date ____________________

Email address ____________________________

Sponsor (Academy Member, Please Print) ____________________________

Sponsor's Signature ____

Date ____________________________

Return application to AAOM, P.O. Box 2016, Edmonds, Washington 980202. Phone: 425.778.6162 **REV 08.18.09**

1. Predental Education ______
   College, dates, and degrees ______
2. Dental and Professional Postdoctoral Education ______
   Schools, dates, and degrees ______
3. Licensed to practice dentistry, date(s), location(s) ______
4. Types of specialty and years in specialty practice ______
5. Are you certified in that specialty? ______ If yes, date certified ______
6. Membership in professional societies ______

______

______

7. Government Service, Military or Civilian (at present, not reserve status)
   (a) Service ______ (b) Rank ______
8. Teaching service in dental, medical or other schools
   (a) Name of School ______
   (b) Title ______
   (c) Subject Taught ______ (d) Date ______
9. Hospital Staff or Services
   Staff Rank ______ Dates ______
10. Research in progress & completed (attach information) ______

______

______

11. Why are you interested in AAOM membership? ______

______

12. Has your license to practice in ANY state or jurisdiction been limited, suspended or revoked?
   ______No ______Yes If yes, please explain on attached sheet.
13. Has your DEA certificate to prescribe controlled substances been investigated, limited, suspended, revoked or restricted in any way or voluntarily or involuntarily been relinquished?
   ______No ______Yes If yes, please explain on attached sheet.
14. Have you privileges in ANY hospital been denied, suspended, reduced, revoked or not renewed or involuntarily been relinquished?
   ______No ______Yes If yes, please explain on attached sheet.
15. Have you had an adverse decision against you in a malpractice action and/or Federal tort claim?
   ______No ______Yes If yes, please explain on attached sheet
16. Have you had any felony criminal convictions?
   ______No ______Yes If yes, please explain on attached sheet.

I attest that the statements in this application are true.

Applicant Signature ______

______

FOR OFFICE USE ONLY Date of Election ______

Action considered by Board (Approved or Tabled) ______ ______

Membership Chair Date

Return application to AAOM, P.O. Box 2016, Edmonds, Washington 980202. Phone: 425.778.6162 REV 08.18.09

Made in United States
Orlando, FL
27 September 2024

52044189R00027